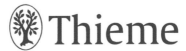

Getting Ready for Brain Tumor Surgery

Michael Sabel, MD
Professor
Department of Neurosurgery
University Hospital Düsseldorf
Düsseldorf, Germany

50 illustrations

Thieme
Stuttgart • New York • Delhi • Rio de Janeiro

Library of Congress Cataloging-in-Publication Data
is available from the publisher.

© 2017 by Georg Thieme Verlag KG
Thieme Publishers Stuttgart
Rüdigerstrasse 14, 70469 Stuttgart, Germany
+49 [0]711 8931 421, customerservice@thieme.de

Thieme Publishers New York
333 Seventh Avenue, New York, NY 10001 USA
+1 800 782 3488, customerservice@thieme.com

Thieme Publishers Delhi
A-12, Second Floor, Sector-2, Noida-201301
Uttar Pradesh, India
+91 120 45 566 00, customerservice@thieme.in

Thieme Publishers Rio, Thieme Publicações Ltda.
Edifício Rodolpho de Paoli, 25º andar
Av. Nilo Peçanha, 50 - Sala 2508
Rio de Janeiro 20020-906 Brasil
+55 21 3172 2297 / +55 21 3172 1896

Cover design: Thieme Publishing Group
Cover Illustration: Mara Gluscak and Renate Diener
Typesetting by DiTech Process Solutions, India

Printed in Germany by CPI Books GmbH

ISBN 978-3-13-240957-6   123456

Also available as an e-book:
eISBN 978-3-13-240999-6

Important note: Medicine is an ever-changing science undergoing continual development. Research and clinical experience are continually expanding our knowledge, in particular our knowledge of proper treatment and drug therapy. Insofar as this book mentions any dosage or application, readers may rest assured that the authors, editors, and publishers have made every effort to ensure that such references are in accordance with **the state of knowledge at the time of production of the book**.

Nevertheless, this does not involve, imply, or express any guarantee or responsibility on the part of the publishers in respect to any dosage instructions and forms of applications stated in the book. **Every user is requested to examine carefully** the manufacturers' leaflets accompanying each drug and to check, if necessary in consultation with a physician or specialist, whether the dosage schedules mentioned therein or the contraindications stated by the manufacturers differ from the statements made in the present book. Such examination is particularly important with drugs that are either rarely used or have been newly released on the market. Every dosage schedule or every form of application used is entirely at the user's own risk and responsibility. The authors and publishers request every user to report to the publishers any discrepancies or inaccuracies noticed. If errors in this work are found after publication, errata will be posted at www.thieme.com on the product description page.

Some of the product names, patents, and registered designs referred to in this book are in fact registered trademarks or proprietary names even though specific reference to this fact is not always made in the text. Therefore, the appearance of a name without designation as proprietary is not to be construed as a representation by the publisher that it is in the public domain.

For Carl and Max. I am very proud of you.

Contents

Preface

This is the first edition of a book that I desperately needed when I was a resident. When you are about to learn one of the most complex professions of the world, you are obviously intimidated when it comes to the action. I remember how insecure I was when I, for the first time, put knife to skin or perforator to skull. My insecurity blocked my performance and prevented me from enjoying the most fascinating profession of the world: Neurosurgery. If someone had shown me that in principle many of the surgical tasks are as simple as preparing a simple meal and brilliant performance is just the result of focused training, it would have been easier for my ego, more effective for the residency program and better for my patients. The crucial difference between simple mechanical tasks in the kitchen and the OR is the fact that the steps you take when preparing dinner are trained for years (cutting, peeling etc.) and are performed in a relaxed mode. In the OR you are unfamiliar with the tasks and not relaxed ... There is an obvious solution: get familiar with the manual tasks in a secure environment where errors don't inflict harm. There is also an ethical aspect involved: why do we train our imperfect manual skills on a patient? Performing subpial dissection first on a patient and not on a cadaver brain? Having your first experience with the microscope during surgery and thereby delaying and slowing down the procedure?

I hope that this book helps to avoid or ameliorate these problems by suggesting simple but still effective training sessions. As you will see: with a little engagement you will be able to train basic skills needed for major aspects of brain tumor surgery.

Michael Sabel

Acknowledgment

I would like to thank all the participants of the "Skills LAB courses" who helped me with their feedback. Thanks also to the residents in the neurosurgery program at the University Hospital Düsseldorf and to Johannes Knipps for his dedicated technical support. Special thanks to our chairman, Prof. H.J. Steiger for his inspiring leadership. Very special thanks to Marion Rapp PhD, MD and Marcel Kamp MD for covering my back and being the best possible colleagues.

Introduction

During the process of becoming a neurosurgeon, many of the necessary skills that need to be acquired can only be mastered by mounting experience during a long-lasting educational progress. However, many (often essential) practical skills can quickly be learned and mastered, depending only on a structured education and focused training. The scope of this book is to provide the young neurosurgeon with a basic set of exercises, which will improve motor skills, handling of tissue, technical competence, and self-confidence. For none of these exercises, a dedicated, expensive, and unpractical laboratory is needed. It is sufficient to have coconuts, chicken wings, bell pepper, agar-agar, a marker pen, and most importantly initiative and motivation. Thus, for many of the exercises, you rather need a grocery shop, than an operating room (OR).

Every hospital can provide you with the rest: battered instruments, unused sutures, cottonoids, etc., are usually discarded. The surgical microscopes are usually not used on weekends; the same applies for the use of a Mayfield clamp or electrical drills. You will not need a dedicated laboratory space; every exercise can (in principle) be performed on your writing desk.

We have defined mental exercises and workstations, which can be all put up either during a dedicated *skills-laboratory day* or as an individual training exercise. We suggest that you find training buddies: it is more fun, more efficient, and (as you might need to purchase some instruments) cheaper. For each chapter, we define the objective, the necessary instruments, and the set-up. We provide a detailed instruction for the set-up and performance of the task by pictures and videos.

1 Planning a Procedure: The Importance of Visualization

This is a very important practical-intellectual exercise.

Relevance for your daily practice

This exercise is highly relevant! The principles described in this exercise will apply for virtually every procedure that you perform.

1.1
Objective

The objective of this chapter is to improve your understanding of a surgical procedure. Understanding is essential to perform.

Visualization

Visualization is the process of creating a mental image of your planned physical action. It is very useful for learning physical exercises (and for what matters surgery is a physical activity).[1]

1.2
You Need

You need paper and pen.

1.3
The Exercise

Start by choosing a simple procedure, which you already have performed or which you (in principle) are able to perform. In your mind, you need to go through every detail of the procedure, including preparation of the surgical theater. Write it down. Be as precise as possible.

1.4
Example

You are going to perform a ventriculostomy (external drainage). Visualize the following points:
- Define your mission statement:
  - At the end of surgery, the drainage needs to produce a free flow of cerebrospinal fluid.
  - You want to position the tip of the drainage in the center of the ventricle, in the direction of the foramen of Monro.
- Check the OR for the instruments which are essential:
  - Do you need ultrasound?
  - Do you need navigation?
  - Check with the nurses, if they are aware of the procedure.
- Visualize the position of the patient.
- Left or right?

- Where do you shave?
- What is the exact position of the burr hole?
- Where is the skin incision?
- Straight or curved incision?
- How do you shave?
- How do you drape?
- Putting the knife to the skin: will you push through to the bone?

We think you got the point: by visualization of the micro-steps you will:

- Identify yet unsolved/not clarified problems (i.e., you plan to use the ultrasound: it is, however, in use and not available; do you place the burr hole on the left or right?).
- You might identify insecurities, which result from your lack of knowledge (where is Kocher's point exactly? In which direction will you insert the drainage?).
  There is no problem, if you do not know things: you are still in the beginning of your education. You are supposed to ask. There is, however, a big problem if you start surgery without knowing exactly where to put the burr hole and if you have only a faint idea in which direction to insert the drainage.
- If your visualization results in a clear mental picture (or movie) of the procedure, you will be quick, precise, and very well organized.

With your growing experience, dedicated visualization will not be necessary for every procedure. However, do not become overconfident: the big mistakes are usually performed by residents who have lost the respect for a (now in their experience very simple) procedure.

Reference

1. Brouziyne M, Molinaro C. Mental imagery combined with physical practice of approach shots for golf beginners. Percept Mot Skills 2005;101(1):203–211

2 The Craniotomy

This is a very practical, simple, and very effective exercise.

Relevance for your daily practice

It is highly relevant! It is the "opener" of brain tumor surgery. Mastering the craniotomy is essential for your integration into the surgical team and burdens you with true responsibility.

2.1
Objective

The objective of this chapter is to improve your practical skills in handling a basic neurosurgical procedure. Guiding a craniotome is in principle a very simple procedure. However, if you have never handled this type of instrument at all, you will feel uncomfortable and unsecure when you perform this for the first time on a patient. You will maneuver this powerful "jigsaw" near to the sinuses and might injure the brain by perforating the dura, observed by an impatient senior surgeon, with time pressure in your back. Therefore, it is best to get some manual experience in a controlled setting.

2.2
You Need

You need a coconut, a mobile drill, craniotome, a Mayfield clamp, a fixation system for the Mayfield clamp (a simple board), and a pen, as well as lots of irrigation and (to spare you a lot of cleaning work) drapes and a bucket, which collects the irrigation/coconut debris.

Ok, we know: you do not own a craniotome and a Mayfield clamp. Here comes your initiative into play. After all, you made it through med school and you made it into a Resident program. Talk to your chief and your head nurse. Explain what you plan to do, especially that you will not work with biological hazardous tissue, which would make the return of the instruments into the OR impossible (i.e., sheep brain).

2.3
The Exercise

Fix the Mayfield clamp to a stable surface (**Fig. 2.1**). Put the coconut into the clamp (**Fig. 2.2**). Set up the perforator or drill. Now, design the planned craniotomy by drawing the outline on the coconut.

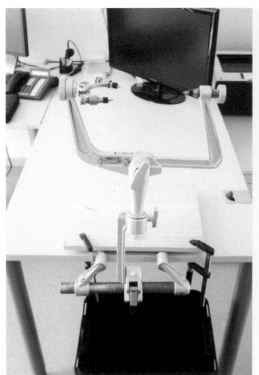

Fig. 2.1 Fixation of the Mayfield clamp to an office desk with screw clamps.

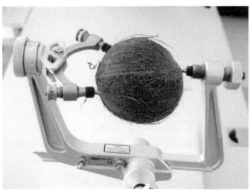

Fig. 2.2 Placement of the coconut in the clamp with marking the outline of the planned craniotomy.

Place the burr hole or work with a drill (**Video 1**; **Fig. 2.3a, b**). Assume that the brownish surface that covers the fruit flesh is the dura mater and should be preserved. Get the feeling for the performance of the perforator and the drill. Take the craniotome and follow the outline (**Video 2**). The point is that you acquire enough

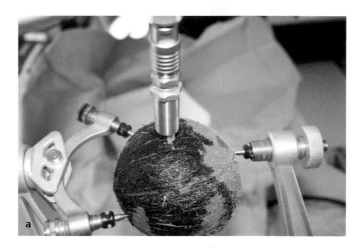

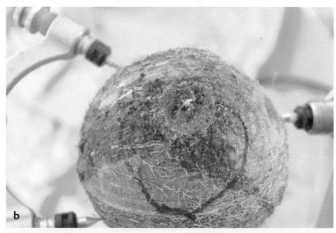

Fig. 2.3 (a, b) Performing the burr hole.

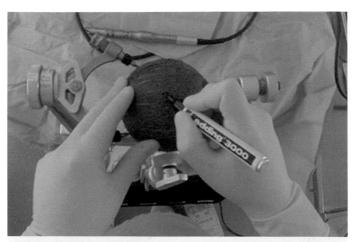

Video 1 Place the burr hole.

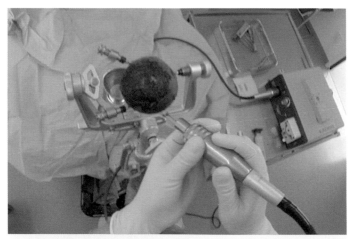

Video 2 Perform the craniotomy.

dexterity to saw out even complex figures (**Fig. 2.4a–c**). You will need lots of irrigation, otherwise the blade will break. You will also understand why water-cooling is important: this very hot metal is very near to essential brain structures.

A coconut is much harder than a human skull and therefore the craniotomy is more difficult. Thus, if "you can make it here and can make it everywhere." Of course, this is not a 100% realistic model, but if you are confident with coconuts, you will feel more confident doing your first craniotomies in the OR.

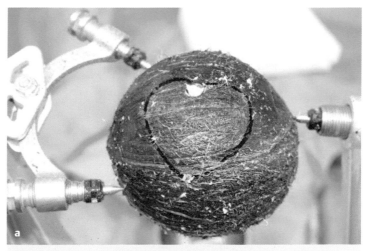

Fig. 2.4 (a–c) Try this on Valentine's day (not on a patient!). (*Continued*)

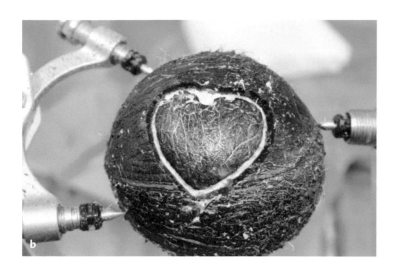

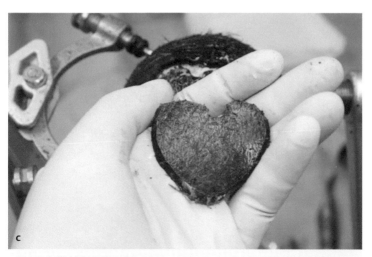

Fig. 2.4 (b, c) (*continued*) Try this on Valentine's day (not on a patient!).

Recommended Readings

Nader R, Costagliola C, Gragnaniello C. Convexity and Parasagittal Approaches. In Nader R, Gragnaniello C, Berta SC, Sabbagh AJ, Levy ML, eds. Neurosurgery Tricks of the Trade: Cranial. New York: Thieme; 2013:2–6

Procedures, interventions, operations: Specific Craniotomies. In: Greenberg MS, ed. Handbook of Neurosurgery. New York: Thieme;2016: 1445–1471

General craniotomy techniques. In: Connolly ES, ed. Fundamentals of Operative Technique in Neurosurgery. New York: Thieme; 2002:196–202

3 Working with the Microscope

This chapter will combine the training of two skills: mastering the microscope and training your bimanual hand coordination. Again, this is a practical, simple, and very effective exercise.

Relevance for your daily practice

This exercise is essential if you work with the microscope. Especially, if you work on deep-seated lesions, this exercise will be very important.

3.1
Objective

The objective of this chapter is to improve your practical skills in using the microscope and coordinating your fine finger and hands movements while using a microscope. There will come a time when you will be asked to take over the microscope and start on your first intracerebral procedure. It would be pretty embarrassing if immediately after taking over the first thing you do is to knock out your assistant with the microscope, get confused with focus and zoom, and show discoordination using suction and bipolar.

Hence, one should:

- Get very familiar with the microscope. A microscope is in principle a very simple instrument. It has less buttons than your remote control at home.
- Get as familiar with the coordination between left hand (i.e., suction) and right hand (i.e., bipolar, forceps) as you are familiar with fork and knife.

3.2
You Need

You need a bell pepper, a plaster, a scalpel, bipolar forceps, biopsy forceps, and a microscope.

As discussed in Chapter 2, ask the relevant persons in your hospital to allow you to work with the microscope. Usually, you will be allowed to move the microscope to an office space near to the OR. If this is not possible, this exercise is entirely feasible in the OR.

3.3
The Exercise

Built a stable stand for the bell pepper by using the plaster stripes (in our case, kindly provided by the Department of Trauma Surgery; **Video 3, Fig. 3.1**).

Make a small incision (maximum 2.5 cm) on the top of the bell pepper and remove the top. Look into the hole: will you be able to take one of the seeds on the bottom without stretching the border of the hole and without damaging the seeds above your target? Is there enough illumination? Your answer should lead you to the need for a microscope.

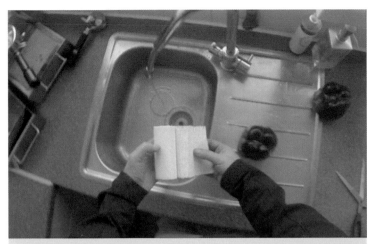

Video 3 Building a stand for the bell pepper.

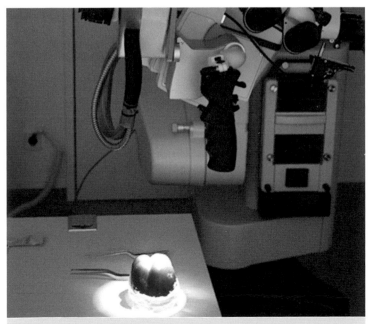

Fig. 3.1 Building a stable support for the bell pepper with plaster rolls.

So, move in the microscope. Now you need to:

- Switch on the microscope. Become familiar with the switches for brake, zoom, and focus. Control the position of the oculars: do you need to correct for your eyesight? Adapt these to your eye distance: you usually do this by looking through the oculars (light switched on, where is this switch?) and adjusting the screws until you have full fusion.

- Establish the correct position of the microscope toward the surgical field. Check that you have the full range of movement of the microscope in this position.

- Balance the microscope: this is obviously dependent on the type of microscope you are using. You need to be familiar with this procedure.

- We strongly recommend that you perform this exercise in a sitting position. Get a chair (any chair will do, but preferably one with variable height), put the chair in position and move in the microscope. Sit down and center the microscope above the bell pepper.

- Find a position that allows for the maximum use of zoom and focus in regard to the target structure: this is your optimal working distance. It is usually 25 cm between lenses and surface. This distance is a given and cannot be changed.

- Based on this position, you will need to settle in. It is essential that you find a position, which is very comfortable and relaxing (**Fig. 3.2a, b**; incorrect and correct positions). Though everybody is very concerned about your wellbeing, this is not the reason why we stress your comfort. You will only be able to perform with your best level of dexterity if your body is not under unnecessary physical strain.

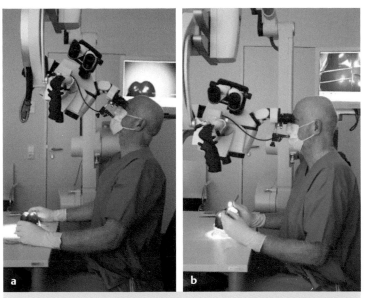

Fig. 3.2 Incorrect (**a**) and correct (**b**) position at the microscope: relax.

- If everything is fine, start exploring the depth of the situs. Move the focus from the surface down to the bottom of the cavity; zoom in and out. Try to explore the depth of the whole cavity (**Fig. 3.3**). To this end you will need to move the corpus of the microscope. With this exercise you will understand the principle of the inverted pyramid (**Fig. 3.4, Video 4**).

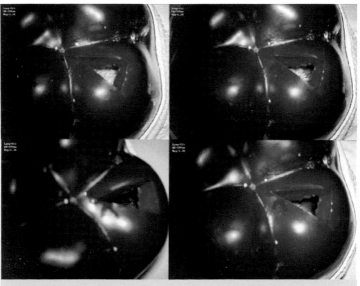

Fig. 3.3 Exploring the depth of the situs by moving the microscope.

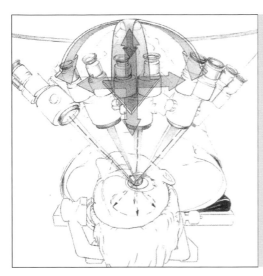

Fig. 3.4 The principle of the inverted pyramid. Despite the small opening, the expert use of the microscope allows for a wide range of visualization. (Used with permission from Yasargil M. Microsurgery: Applied to Neurosurgery. New York, NY: Thieme; 2006.)

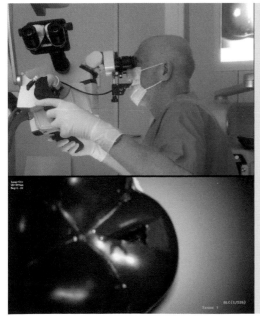

Video 4 The principle of the inverted pyramid.

Now you are ready to start surgery. Take the bipolar in your left and the forceps in your right hand and start to pick out the seeds. Get familiar with this and then gradually increase the difficulty: pick out a seed without touching the surface, without touching other seeds, etc. (**Fig. 3.5, Video 5**). You will often block your field of view by your own hands (**Fig. 3.6**). Try to avoid this. Remember that the tip of your sharp instrument is deeply inserted in a brain—you absolutely need visual control.

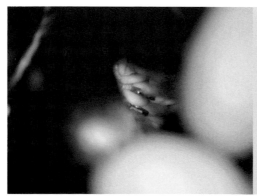

Fig. 3.5 Choose a seed and try to grip it precisely.

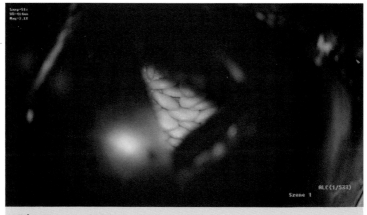

Video 5 Removal of the seeds.

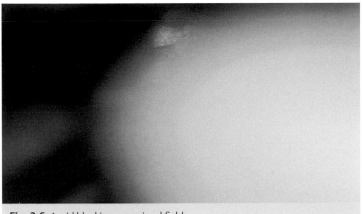

Fig. 3.6 Avoid blocking your visual field.

Recommended Reading

Levy ML, Berta S. General and advanced cranial approaches: 5—
Interhemispheric transcallosal transchoroidal approach to the
third ventricle. In Nader R, Gragnaniello C, Berta SC, Sabbagh
AJ, Levy ML, eds. Neurosurgery Tricks of the Trade: Cranial.
New York: Thieme; 2013:19–22

4 Removing a Gyrus: The Principle of Subpial Resection

This chapter will introduce you into tissue handling at an already quite sophisticated level. However, if you understand the principle of this technique already at an early stage of your training, you will be more capable of understanding the surgery in which you will only assist during your first years. In this chapter, you will learn how to remove a gyrus, a technique essential in resection of infiltrating tumors. At the same time, you will learn some important anatomical lessons.

Relevance for your daily practice

The understanding of this resection technique is of utmost importance for high-level brain tumor surgery.

4.1 Objective

The objective of this chapter is to give you a basic understanding of the principles of brain tissue removal.

Imagine the following scenario: imagine that you plan to resect a low-grade glioma, which for the major part (according to magnetic resonance imaging) is superficially located in a gyrus (**Fig. 4.1**). Due to the biology of the tumor, you need to assume that large parts of the gyrus are infiltrated by tumor cells. You have tested the functionality of the gyrus by neuromonitoring.[1–3] According to your findings, the tumor harboring gyrus can be removed. Your task is now to remove this gyrus without damaging the adjacent gyri, in which (unfortunately) you have located the motor functions. Please review and understand the anatomy of this situation by studying the illustration (**Fig. 4.2**). Note the pial layer which cover the surface of the brain. You will have to cut through this layer using a scissor or knife. This layer offers protection for the underlying structures and therefore also for the vessel running in the sulcus (**Fig. 4.2**) and the adjacent brain. If you

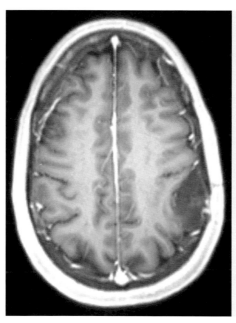

Fig 4.1 Low-grade glioma, in the superior parts confined to the extensions of the gyrus.

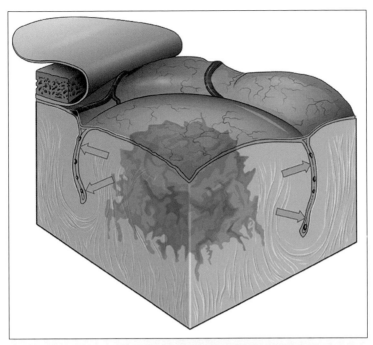

Fig. 4.2 Schematic drawing of an infiltrating brain tumor. Note the pial confinement.

manage to remove the brain without perforating the pia, these structures are relatively safe. This surgical technique is called subpial resection. Apart from safety issues, this technique implies (in the area of subpial coverage) a complete biological resection of the tumor (*no brain, no tumor*). Please realize that as soon you enter the white matter at the bottom of the gyrus, the situation changes: you might enter functional fiber tracts, so your resection technique needs to change. Let us, however, focus on the subpial resection for the moment.

As you will have deducted from the above, you need a brain (to train on ☺). It needs to be fresh and have in principle the same anatomical features as a human one. Problem? No, not at all. At least in Germany, France, and Spain, sheep brains are regularly used for cooking and available in supermarkets or (in Germany) in Turkish grocery shops. The best thing is sheep brains are cheap. You will not spend more than €2 per brain. If you have absolutely no access to sheep brains, call a local slaughterhouse: they will be able to provide you with pig or cow brain (approximately €3).

There is, however, one disadvantage with this material: for obvious reasons you are absolutely not allowed to use instruments that might cycle back to the OR! Therefore, get your separate set of instruments. We have included pictures of typical instruments you will need. You can easily order these in the Internet. All in all, this will put you back for €200 max. However, as mentioned earlier, your hospital is certainly capable of providing you with instruments that need replacement. As brain tissue is preferably removed with suction, you should try to organize a suction device. As this exercise is not feasible in the OR, you need to use an electric suction pump. If your hospital is not equipped with electrical vacuum pumps, you will need to improvise. We successfully build a vacuum pump by converting an aquarium pump. If you are able to spend a little money, electric pumps for medical use are available in the Internet (approximately €240). Do not worry if you do not manage to procure suction: the point of this exercise is to understand the principle of resection.

4.2
You Need

Fresh sheep brain, scalpel no. 11, micro-dissector, micro-hook, microscope, electric suction, and micro-forceps are required (**Fig. 4.3**).

As this exercise is not feasible in the OR, you will need to find a suitable room: any office will do.

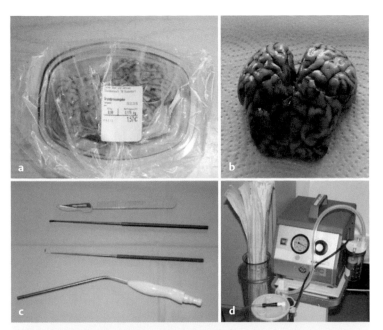

Fig. 4.3 Sheep brains are cheap. There are only few instruments necessary. It is important to have a suction available.

4.3
The Exercise

There are two variants of this exercise: either you use the mic or you perform this exercise macroscopically. If you are already an advanced user of the mic, you should try the variant without mic: it is a valuable lesson, as you might realize that for the resection of superficial lesions the mic is not essential. To the contrary, your technique might even benefit from the improved anatomical overview. Most of you, however, will benefit from the use of the mic. This chapter includes all the features of Chapter 3.

Put the brain on a suitable surface.

- Switch on the mic, remember and put into practice what you have learned in Chapter 3.
- Choose a gyrus that you want to resect. Your mission is to completely resect that gyrus and completely preserve the adjacent gyri. This includes the pial surface!
- Enter the "chosen one" by opening the pia with the knife (**Fig. 4.3**).

Exercise A (**Video 6**)

- Use the dissector to mobilize the cortex from the pia (**Fig. 4.4**).

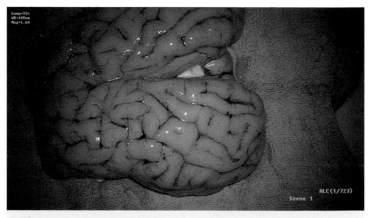

Video 6 Opening a gyrus. Mobilizing the cortex by separation from pia. Removal of tissue up to the next pial border.

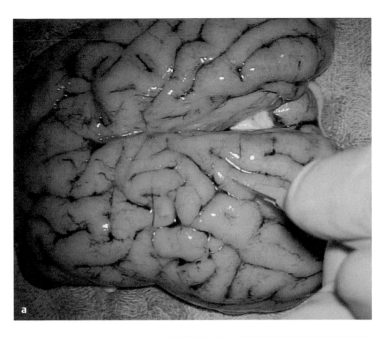

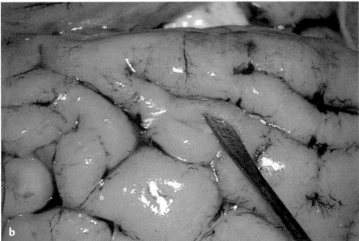

Fig. 4.4 Mobilize the cortex from the pia.

- Stay below the pial layer (**Fig. 4.5**).
- Remove the mobilized tissue with the forceps (**Fig. 4.6**).
- Try to identify the sulcal anatomy: where is the pia and where is the adjacent gyrus?
- Is the adjacent gyrus damaged?
- Is the target gyrus completely removed?
- Assess the damage.

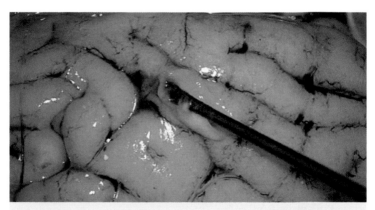

Fig. 4.5 Stay below the pial layer.

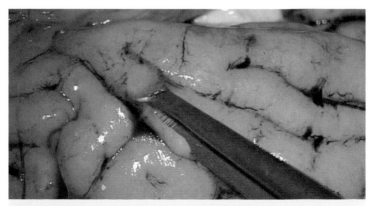

Fig. 4.6 Remove the mobilized tissue with the forceps.

You will realize that you need to exert substantial force on the adjacent gyri and that you will pull out the tissue with some force. There is a better technique.

Exercise B (**Video 6**)

- Use the bipolar with spreading movements to mobilize the tissue.
- Now take the suction and remove the mobilized tissue (**Fig. 4.7**).
- Remove the adjacent, not mobilized tissue.
- Work with different suction strengths.
- Assess the damage.
- You need to see an undamaged "next" gyrus. This is the end point of this exercise (**Fig. 4.8**).

It is important that you get the feeling for the different resection techniques. For motivation, imagine that the patient is awake and that every manipulation of the adjacent gyri is inducing a temporary speech arrest.

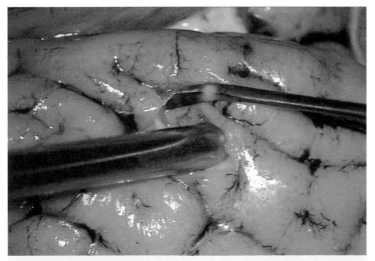

Fig. 4.7 Take the suction and remove the mobilized tissue.

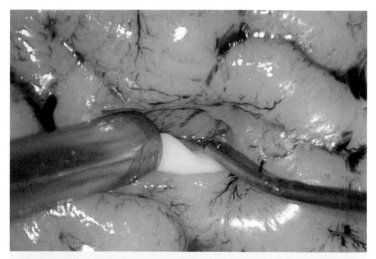

Fig. 4.8 You need to see an undamaged "next" gyrus. This is the end point of this exercise.

References

1. Duffau H. Resecting diffuse low-grade gliomas to the boundaries of brain functions: a new concept in surgical neuro-oncology. J Neurosurg Sci 2015;59(4):361–371
2. Duffau H. A new concept of diffuse (low-grade) glioma surgery. Adv Tech Stand Neurosurg 2012;38:3–27
3. Gil-Robles S, Duffau H. Surgical management of World Health Organization Grade II gliomas in eloquent areas: the necessity of preserving a margin around functional structures. Neurosurg Focus 2010;28(2):E8

Recommended Reading

Duffau H, ed. New insights into the therapeutic strategies for DLGG: Surgery for diffuse low-grade gliomas. In: Diffuse Low-Grade Gliomas in Adults. New York: Springer;2013:359–374

5 Removing an Artificial Brain Tumor

This chapter is obviously based on Chapter 4. Refining your technique to remove normal brain tissue is important, but not really the crucial point in brain tumor surgery. Hence, in this chapter you will be trained to remove tissue with a different consistency (we make it harder for you) with the option to get your first experience with fluorescence-guided surgery.[1]

Relevance for your daily practice

If you are starting to work on brain tumors, you will find this lesson very relevant, as it increases your dexterity in handling pathological tissue.

5.1
Objective

The objective of this chapter is to train your dexterity in removing pathological tissue.

In this chapter, we take your experience from Chapter 4 a little further. You will remove a brain tumor: actually it is not a brain tumor, but a lump of agar-agar. The crucial point is that in this scenario gentle suction and manipulation of the tissue will not be efficient. You will need to increase the force that you apply. On the other hand, rules from chapter 4 apply: you are very near to crucial, highly functional tissue.

5.2
You Need

You need set-up from Chapter 4 plus agar-agar, boiling water, a pink marker pen, and syringe with large bore needle (**Fig. 5.1**), as well as ultrasound (if available) and microscope with blue-light equipment.

As in Chapter 4, this exercise is not feasible in the OR.

For this chapter, you need to prepare the brains first. It will take less than 5 minutes, so you can do this before you start the exercise.

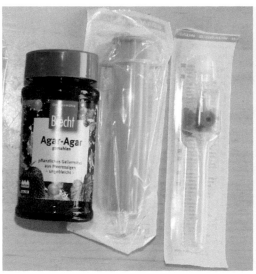

Fig. 5.1 In addition to the equipment of Chapter 4, you need a marker pen and a large bore needle with syringe.

5.3
The Exercise

Preparation of the brain tumor: You can do this the day before, that is, at your home (see **Video 7**). Dissolve two tablespoons of agar-agar in 50 mL of warm water in a pan; bring it to the boiling point and then let the solution cool down. Put in some drops of the highlighter ink, and stir and aspirate into syringe. Now you need to be relatively quick: the solution might harden within a couple of minutes. Carefully inject 2 to 3 mL with a large bore

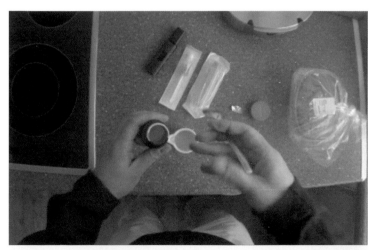

Video 7 Preparation of the artificial brain tumor.

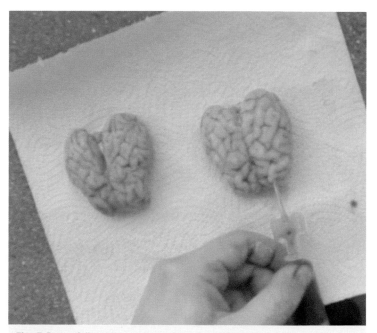

Fig. 5.2 Carefully inject 2 to 3 mL of the mass using the large bore needle into the brain. Use a tangential approach; otherwise the clot will be injected into the ventricles.

needle into the brain. Use a tangential approach; otherwise the clot will be injected into the ventricles (**Fig. 5.2**, **Video 7**).

By variation of the concentration, you will end up with different consistencies and colorization.

This chapter includes all the features of Chapters 3 and 4.

Put the brain on a suitable surface.

- Do you remember where you injected the tumor? You might see the tumor reaching the surface.
- If available, try to identify the tumor with ultrasound (**Fig. 5.3**, **Video 8**). We find this a very useful technique to train the use of ultrasound. Remember that you absolutely need to cover the ultrasound probe.

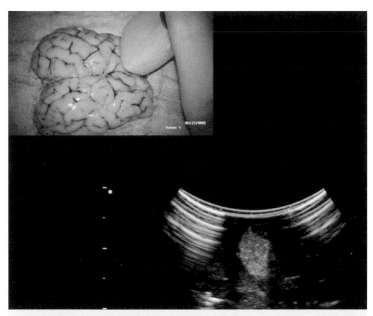

Fig. 5.3 Identification of the tumor with ultrasound.

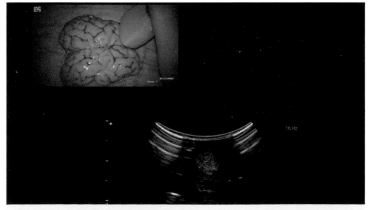

Video 8 Identification of the tumor by ultrasound.

- Switch on the mic. Check for fluorescence by switching on blue light (**Fig. 5.4a, b**). Remember and put into practice what you have learned in Chapters 3 and 4.

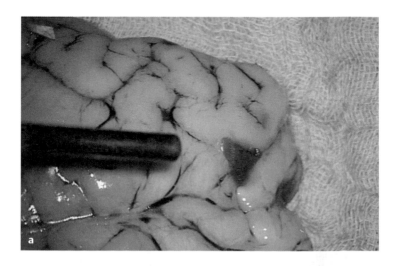

Fig. 5.4 (a, b) Check for fluorescence by switching on blue light.

- Open the gyrus in which you suspect the tumor. Your mission is to resect the tumor completely and to preserve the adjacent gyri as trained in Chapter 4 (**Fig. 4.8**).
- Work with dissector (**Fig. 5.5**) or hook. Try to mobilize the tumor. Work with suction and hook or dissector (**Fig. 5.6, Video 9**).

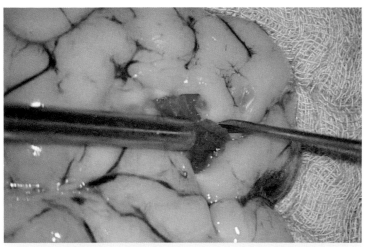

Fig. 5.5 Work with dissector or hook. Try to mobilize the tumor.

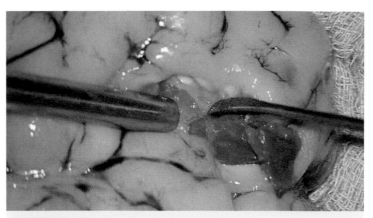

Fig. 5.6 Work with suction and hook or dissector.

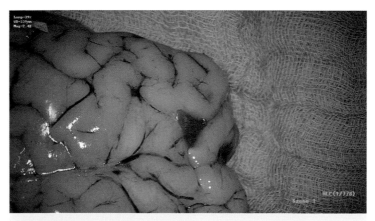

Video 9 Resection of the tumor.

- If you have resected the major parts of the tumor, check for residual fluorescence (**Fig. 5.7**).

It is important that you get the feeling for the different resection techniques. For motivation, imagine that the sheep (ups) patient is awake and that every manipulation of the adjacent gyri is inducing a temporary speech arrest.

Fig. 5.7 Check for residual fluorescence.

Reference

1. Kamp MA, Knipps J, Steiger HJ, et al. Training for brain tumour resection: a realistic model with easy accessibility. Acta Neurochir (Wien) 2015;157(11):1975–1981, discussion 1981

Recommended Readings

Hassaneen W, Sawaya R. General and advanced cranial approaches: 16—Glioma resection. In Nader R, Gragnaniello C, Berta SC, Sabbagh AJ, Levy ML, eds. Neurosurgery Tricks of the Trade: Cranial. New York: Thieme; 2013

Duffau H, ed. Part VI 23 Surgery for Diffuse Low-Grade Gliomas. In: Diffuse Low-Grade Gliomas in Adults. New York: Springer

Gil-Robles S, Duffau H. Surgical management of World Health Organization Grade II gliomas in eloquent areas: the necessity of preserving a margin around functional structures. Neurosurg Focus 2010;28(2):E8

6 Microsurgical Training: The Chicken Wing Model

This chapter trains your fine finger movements. In the previous chapters, we focused on planning, coordination, and rougher motor skills. With this exercise, we will expose you to microsurgery and your tremor. Unfortunately, microsurgery is often mystified as an elite field, which requires special gifts. There will of course be a small population of especially gifted people around us, but believe me, with motivation, some endurance, good teaching, and training, nearly everybody will be able to perform complicated microsurgical procedures. You can prove this to yourself by suturing a vessel with a diameter of less than 1 mm. No microvascular laboratory? No animal house? No instruments? No problem.

You just need five instruments, sutures, and a chicken wing.[1]

Relevance for your daily practice

Suturing small vessel is of virtually no practical relevance for your daily practice. However, the confidence in your skills that you will achieve by practicing with this model is very valuable and will support you if you (and that will happen) question your principle skills. On the other hand, maybe you will become so fascinated with this kind of surgery that you will become very interested in cerebral bypass surgery.

6.1
Objective

The objective of this exercise is to train your fine finger movements, provide you with confidence that you can do microsurgery, and test and train your endurance.

6.2
You Need

You need chicken wing, Dumont watchmaker forceps no. 5, surgical scissor 10.5 cm or scalpel no. 11, micro-scissor, 6.0–9.0 sutures, and needle holder (**Fig. 6.1**). These instruments are (if not available through your hospital) easy to order via the Internet (total costs around €200). You also need a microscope.

This exercise is feasible in the OR or in any office equipped with a microscope.

6.3
The Exercise
Video 10

Step 1

The setup of your workstation is possible in the OR or in any office where in which you can place a microscope. A table and a chair with adjustable height are important. Also take care to choose a table that is stable and provides enough place for a comfortable rest of your hands and underarms.

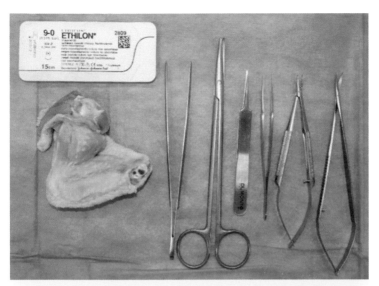

Fig. 6.1 Chicken wing, Dumont watchmaker forceps no. 5, surgical scissor 10.5 cm or scalpel no. 11, micro-scissor, 6.0–9.0 sutures, and needle holder.

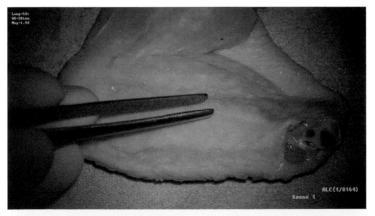

Video 10 Placing a knot with 9.0 sutures in the chicken wing model.

Step 2

Adjust the heights of table and chair to reach a position of maximal relaxation and comfortable positioning of your underarms and wrists (**Fig. 6.2**).

Step 3

Put the chicken wing on a suitable surface. We recommend using a board, which makes rotation of the surgical field easier. Make sure that the board is large enough to accommodate your forearms and especially the wrists.

The brachial artery runs between the palpable muscle bulks. Open the skin with the surgical scissor (**Fig. 6.3a, b**) in the direction of the assumed vessel course and separate the muscle bulks with blunt dissection. You will find the vessel bundle at the bottom of the sulcus.

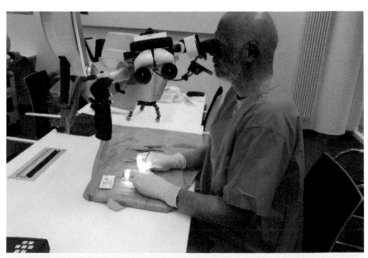

Fig. 6.2 Position of maximal relaxation and comfortable positioning of your underarms and wrists.

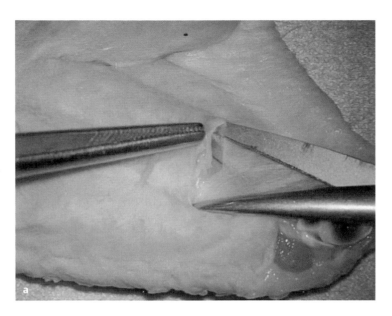

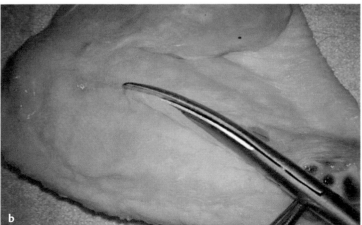

Fig. 6.3 (a, b) The brachial artery runs between the palpable muscle bulks. Open the skin with the surgical scissor.

Step 4

The nerve vessel structures run, interconnected by connective tissue fibers, below a fascia.

Use the microscope and expose the vessel by first opening the fascia. Then, start separating the vascular structures.

Lift the interconnecting tissue with a forceps and cut with the scissor, thus creating a small hole (**Fig. 6.4**).

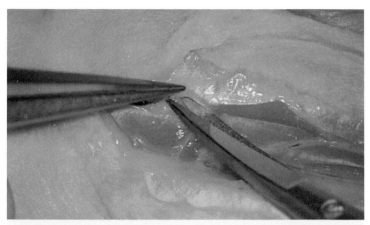

Fig. 6.4 Lift the interconnecting tissue with a forceps and cut with the scissor, thus creating a small hole.

Step 5

Insert a scissor blade into the opening and cut the tissue in parallel to the vessel.

Separate the artery completely from the vein by blunt lateral and longitudinal movements of the closed and intermittently spread forceps or scissors (**Fig. 6.5**).

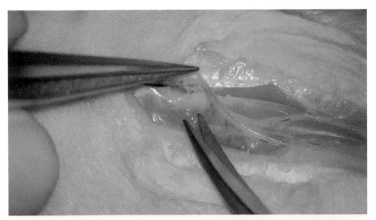

Fig. 6.5 Separate the artery completely from the vein by blunt lateral and longitudinal movements of the closed and intermittently spread forceps or scissors.

Step 6

Proceed until you have performed a complete separation of the artery from the surrounding tissue on a length of at least 5 mm. Put a sheet (piece of rubber glove) between the vessels, thus creating a working surface (**Fig. 6.6a, b**).

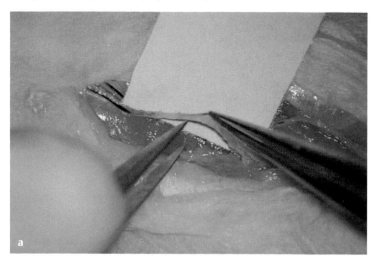

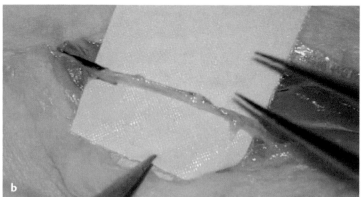

Fig. 6.6 (a, b) Put a sheet (piece of rubber glove) between the vessels, thus creating a working surface.

Step 7

Separate the remaining adventitia from the vessel (**Fig. 6.7**).

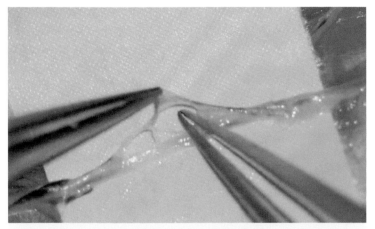

Fig. 6.7 Separate the remaining adventitia from the vessel.

Step 8

Preparing the suture:

Start with a 9.0 suture. Position the styropor block below the microscope. Remove the needle with a needle holder. Position the needle near your surgical situs, within your visual fields (**Fig. 6.8a, b**).

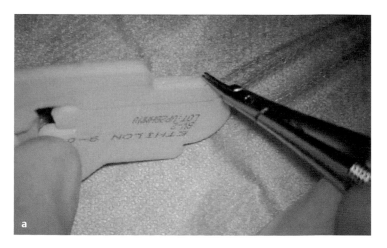

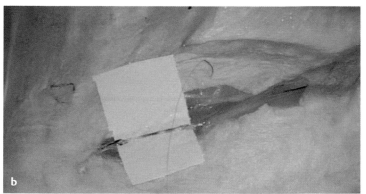

Fig. 6.8 (a, b) Position the needle near your surgical situs, within your visual fields.

Step 9

Cut with one stroke of the micro-scissor perpendicular to the vessel (**Fig. 6.9**).

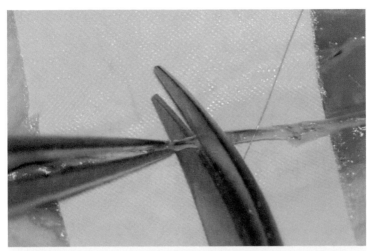

Fig. 6.9 Cut with one stroke of the micro-scissor perpendicular to the vessel.

Step 10

It will help you to position the chicken wing to have the vessel running (diagonally) from your right-upper to your left-lower visual field. Insert the first stitch on the side of your dominant hand. Lift the vessel with the forceps, grasping the adventitia. Insert the needle approximately at the distance of one vessel diameter, perpendicular to the surface and gently push through (**Fig. 6.10**). Grasp the tip of the needle with the dumont 5.

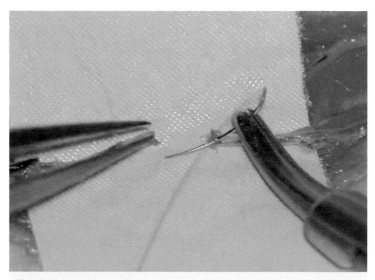

Fig. 6.10 Insert the needle approximately at the distance of one vessel diameter, perpendicular to the surface and gently push through.

Step 11

When the needle has completely passed the vessel, reposition the needle in the needle holder, lift the vessel stump with the forceps, and insert the needle through the vessel lumen, again approximately one diameter behind the lumen (**Fig. 6.11**).

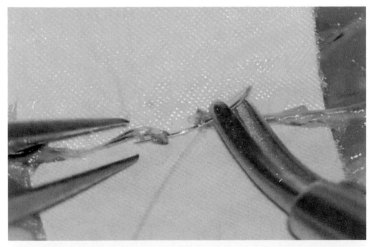

Fig. 6.11 Insert the needle through the vessel lumen, again approximately one diameter behind the lumen.

Step 12

Now draw the suture with a continuous movement through the vessel. Use the tip of a forceps on the vessel to exert a little counterpressure. This will prevent the tearing or torsion of the vessel (**Fig. 6.12**).

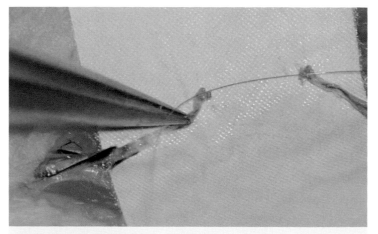

Fig. 6.12 Use the tip of a forceps on the vessel to exert a little counterpressure. This will prevent the tearing or torsion of the vessel.

Step 13

Draw the suture through, until you still have approximately three times the vessel lumen to the end of the suture. This is an ideal rest to grasp when you now perform the first knot. Shorten the suture (**Fig. 6.13**).

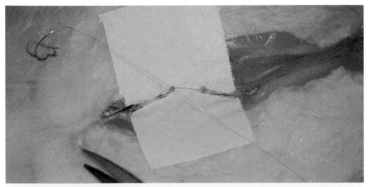

Fig. 6.13 Shorten the suture.

Step 14

The first knot is placed as backhand knot with two loops (**Fig. 6.14**). Gently approximate the stumps—"approximate, do not strangulate" (**Fig. 6.15**). Position one counterknot. Cut the suture. Your first knot is done! Do not expect a perfect result. However, look at the dimensions of the tissue you have just manipulated (**Fig. 6.16**).

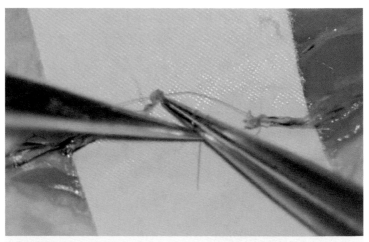

Fig. 6.14 The first knot is placed as backhand knot with two loops.

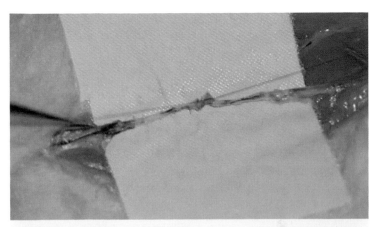

Fig. 6.15 Gently approximate the stumps—"approximate, do not strangulate." Position one counterknot. Cut the suture.

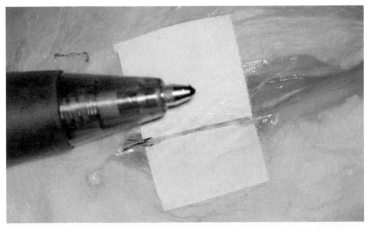

Fig. 6.16 Dimensions of the tissue you have just manipulated.

Reference

1. Hino A. Training in microvascular surgery using a chicken wing artery. Neurosurgery 2003;52(6):1495–1497, discussion 1497–1498

Recommended Reading

Yasargil MG, ed. Microneurosurgery. [Revised Edition] Stuttgart, Germany: Thieme; 1996. Microneurosurgery of CNS Tumors; vol. IVb

Bibliography

Yasargil MG, ed. Microneurosurgery. [Revised Edition] Stuttgart, Germany: Thieme; 1996. Microneurosurgery of CNS Tumors; vol. IVb

Nader R, Gragnaniello C, Berta SC, Sabbagh AJ, Levy ML. Neurosurgery Tricks of the Trade: Cranial. New York: Thieme; 2013

Greenberg MS. Handbook of Neurosurgery. New York, NY: Thieme Medical Publishers; 2016

Duffau H. Diffuse Low-Grade Gliomas in Adults. New York, NY: Springer; 2013

Connolly P. Fundamentals of Operative Technique in Neurosurgery. New York, NY: Thieme Medical Publishers; 2002

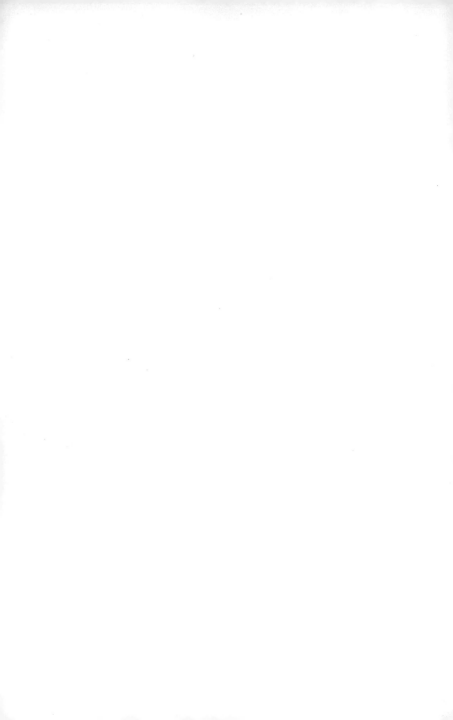